I0436621

HEALING ULCERS NATURALLY

A Comprehensive Guide To Effective Ulcer Therapy

Explore Holistic Approaches And Cutting-Edge Treatments To Combat Ulcers And Promote Lasting Relief

JAMES JOSEPH

CHAPTER ONE

Introduction

Ulcers, which are painful sores that form on the lining of the digestive system, may have a substantial influence on a person's quality of life. These bothersome sores may appear in a variety of digestive organs, including the stomach and small intestine. Understanding the many forms, causes, and symptoms of ulcers is critical for their successful management and treatment. Furthermore, using a holistic approach that includes dietary changes and the use of herbal medicines might help promote healing and relieve ulcer-related symptoms.

Understand Ulcers: Types, Causes, And Symptoms

To understand how to properly treat ulcers, you must first grasp the many kinds, causes, and symptoms of the ailment. Ulcers are classified into two types: gastric ulcers, which grow in the stomach lining, and duodenal ulcers, which form in the upper region of the small intestine known as the duodenum.

The bacteria Helicobacter pylori is a frequent cause of ulcers. This bacteria weakens the stomach and small intestine's protective mucous layer, causing stomach acid to damage the delicate lining underneath. Furthermore, long-term use of nonsteroidal anti-inflammatory medicines (NSAIDs) like aspirin and ibuprofen might cause ulcer development by irritating the stomach lining.

Ulcer symptoms might vary, but some frequent markers include abdominal burning or discomfort, bloating, nausea, and, in severe instances, vomiting. Some people may suffer appetite fluctuations and unintentional weight reduction.

Recognizing these signs is critical for timely diagnosis and action.

The Role of Diet in Ulcer Formation

Ulcer formation and control are heavily influenced by one's diet. While certain meals may aggravate symptoms, others might help the healing process. Individuals with ulcers are often recommended to avoid spicy meals, acidic foods, and caffeinated drinks since they might irritate the stomach lining and promote acid production. Smoking and alcohol intake may further worsen ulcer symptoms and slow the healing process.

On the other hand, eating a diet rich in certain nutrients and avoiding possible triggers may help with ulcer care. Fiber-rich meals, such as fruits, vegetables, and whole grains, may aid digestion and improve gut health. Incorporating lean proteins, probiotics, and low-fat dairy products may also help to maintain a healthy diet and prevent ulcers.

Powerful Healing Foods: A Nutritional Approach To Ulcer Treatment

Certain foods include therapeutic characteristics that may help manage and alleviate ulcer-related symptoms. Individuals with ulcers may consider introducing the following effective healing foods into their diets:

1. Honey is known for its antibacterial and anti-inflammatory characteristics, which may help soothe and cure ulcerated tissues. Manuka honey, in particular, has been investigated for its possible therapeutic effects in H. Helicobacter pylori infections.

2. Aloe Vera: Aloe vera has long been known for its therapeutic powers. It may assist in calming inflamed tissues and decrease inflammation in the digestive

system. Aloe vera juice, when drunk in moderation, may help with ulcer control.

3. Cabbage Juice: Cabbage contains chemicals that may preserve the stomach lining and aid healing. Fresh cabbage juice has been studied as a natural cure for ulcers.

4. Turmeric contains curcumin, which has anti-inflammatory and antioxidant effects. Consuming turmeric or taking turmeric pills may aid in ulcer healing.

5. Garlic contains antibacterial and anti-inflammatory qualities that may help treat ulcers. It is best to eat garlic in moderation, since excessive use may aggravate symptoms in certain people.

6. Ginger, known for its anti-nausea and anti-inflammatory effects, maybe a calming addition to an ulcer-friendly diet. Consider drinking ginger tea or incorporating raw ginger into your meals.

7. Fermented foods such as yogurt, kefir, and sauerkraut include probiotics, which help to maintain a healthy balance of intestinal flora. Probiotics may improve digestive health and may benefit ulcer care.

Individual reactions to these foods may vary, so people with ulcers should speak with a healthcare provider or a certified dietitian before making substantial dietary adjustments.

Herbal Remedies For Ulcers: Leveraging Nature's Healing Potential

In addition to dietary changes, herbal therapies have been investigated for their ability to treat ulcers. While it is important to explore herbal remedies with caution and under the supervision of a healthcare professional, several herbs have shown promise in promoting ulcer healing:

1. Licorice Root: Licorice root includes chemicals that may induce mucus production, so providing a protective layer to the stomach lining. DGL (deglycyrrhizinated licorice) pills are often prescribed to reduce the risks associated with excessive licorice eating.

2. Chamomile: Chamomile contains anti-inflammatory and anti-spasmodic qualities, making it a useful tool for controlling ulcer symptoms. Chamomile tea, in particular, may assist in easing the digestive system.

3. Mastic Gum: Derived from the resin of the mastic tree, mastic gum possesses antibacterial characteristics and has been investigated for its potential in treating H. Helicobacter pylori infections.

4. Slippery Elm is noted for its mucilage content, which creates a calming and protective covering over inflamed tissues. It may be taken in the form of supplements or tea.

5. Marshmallow Root: Like slippery elm, marshmallow root includes mucilage, which helps calm and protect the stomach wall. Marshmallow root tea is a popular preparation.

Herbal treatments should be used with care since they may interfere with drugs or other health issues. It is recommended that you consult with a healthcare practitioner before introducing herbal supplements into your ulcer treatment regimen.

Ulcers may have a substantial influence on an individual's well-being, but with a holistic approach that includes an awareness of the kinds, causes, and symptoms of ulcers, as well as dietary changes and the potential use of herbal treatments, successful management, and alleviation are possible. Adopting a well-balanced and ulcer-friendly diet that is high in healing nutrients and low in possible triggers may help the healing process significantly. Furthermore, when taken correctly and under expert supervision, herbal medicines may provide further help in treating ulcer symptoms and supporting overall digestive health. Individuals suffering from ulcer symptoms should seek immediate medical assistance for the correct diagnosis and specific treatment regimens, just as they would for any other health problem.

CHAPTER TWO

Stress Reduction Methods For Ulcer Healing

Stress has long been recognized as an important element in the development and progression of ulcers. Individuals suffering from stomach or peptic ulcers must manage stress to recover effectively. Stress reduction tactics not only improve mental health but also help with physical healing.

Mindfulness meditation is an excellent stress-reduction strategy. Mindfulness is being present at the moment, concentrating on the breath, and growing awareness without judgment. Numerous studies have shown the beneficial effects of mindfulness on stress reduction and general wellness. Ulcer sufferers may benefit from adopting mindfulness meditation into their everyday routines to reduce stress and promote recovery.

Progressive muscular relaxation is another effective stress-reduction approach. PMR consists of systematically tensing and then releasing various muscle groups in the body. This approach relieves physical tension, which may aid in stress reduction. Ulcer sufferers who practice PMR daily might feel more relaxed, creating an atmosphere favorable to ulcer healing.

The Significance Of Proper Hydration In Ulcer Therapy

Hydration is essential in ulcer treatment because it affects overall gastrointestinal health and aids in the healing process. Proper hydration is necessary for preserving the stomach's mucosal lining and encouraging mucus production, which protects against the corrosive effects of stomach acids.

Water, in particular, is essential for neutralizing stomach acids and avoiding excessive acidity in the stomach. Ulcer sufferers are recommended to drink plenty of water throughout the day to be well-hydrated. Caffeinated and carbonated drinks should be consumed in moderation since they might lead to increased stomach acidity and discomfort.

In addition to water, ulcer sufferers may benefit from drinking herbal teas such as chamomile or ginger tea. These teas are anti-inflammatory and can help calm the digestive system. Including a range of hydrating foods with high water content in your diet, such as watermelon and cucumber, may also help with general hydration and ulcer healing.

Gut Health And Ulcers: Probiotics And Prebiotics For Healing

People with ulcers must maintain a healthy mix of intestinal flora. Probiotics, or helpful bacteria, may help to improve gut health and promote ulcer healing. Consuming probiotic-rich foods like yogurt, kefir, and fermented vegetables can help restore intestinal flora balance.

Prebiotics, on the other hand, are indigestible fibers that provide food for beneficial gut bacteria. Including prebiotic-rich foods in your diet, such as bananas, garlic, and onions, can help probiotics work better and promote a healthier gut environment.

Individuals with ulcers should check with their healthcare professionals before adding probiotics or prebiotics to their diet, since individual reactions may vary. Nonetheless, when combined with competent supervision, these substances may play an important role in gut health and ulcer healing.

Physical Activities For Ulcer Patients: Balancing Exercise With Recovery

Regular physical activity is essential for overall health, including for people who have ulcers. However, finding the correct balance between activity and rest is critical to avoiding unnecessary stress on the body and exacerbating ulcer symptoms.

Low-impact workouts, such as walking, swimming, or moderate yoga, may help ulcer sufferers. These exercises improve blood circulation, digestion, and general well-being while putting little burden on the digestive system. Individuals with ulcers should avoid high-impact and rigorous workouts since they may cause pain or exacerbate their condition.

Incorporating regular, moderate exercise into a daily regimen may help to reduce stress and improve mental health, which aids in the overall healing process. However, any fitness plan should be evaluated by a healthcare practitioner to verify it is appropriate for the individual's unique health condition and requirements.

Sleep And Restorative Practices For Ulcer Relief.

Adequate and quality sleep is crucial for the body's healing and recovery processes, and this holds for persons with ulcers. Sleep enables the body to repair and renew tissues, including the mucosal lining of the stomach, aiding ulcer healing.

Establishing a consistent sleep schedule, keeping a pleasant sleep environment, and practicing relaxation methods before bedtime are vital for ensuring restful sleep. Avoiding stimulants like coffee close to bedtime and maintaining a peaceful and dark resting place might boost the quality of sleep for those with ulcers.

In addition to appropriate sleep, implementing restorative techniques such as deep breathing exercises or mild stretching may further assist in relaxation and stress reduction. These activities contribute to an overall feeling of well-being, which is beneficial to the healing process.

In conclusion, a holistic approach to ulcer care comprises not only medicinal interventions but also lifestyle alterations that promote the body's natural healing processes. Stress reduction measures, sufficient hydration, attention to gut health, balanced physical activity, and prioritizing relaxation and sleep together contribute to establishing an environment favorable to ulcer healing. Individuals with ulcers should work in partnership with healthcare providers to adjust these techniques to their unique requirements and situations, encouraging a holistic and personalized approach to ulcer management.

The mind and body are inextricably linked, and this connection is critical in comprehensive ulcer treatment. Ulcers, whether gastric or peptic, may entail a complicated interaction of physical, emotional, and psychological variables. Recognizing and treating the mind-body link may make a substantial contribution to a holistic treatment plan.

CHAPTER THREE

Mind-Body Connection: A Holistic Approach To Ulcer Healing

Holistic methods of ulcer healing highlight the necessity of taking into account both mental and physical well-being. Stress, for example, has been implicated as a component in the development and progression of ulcers. The body's stress reaction causes the production of hormones and chemicals that might harm the digestive tract, thereby exacerbating ulcer symptoms.

Mindfulness approaches, such as meditation and deep breathing exercises, have shown potential in stress reduction and mental health promotion. Incorporating these activities throughout everyday life may help to promote a more balanced mind-body connection, possibly reducing the influence of stress on ulcer disorders.

Furthermore, holistic treatment often entails maintaining a healthy lifestyle, which includes a well-balanced diet, regular exercise, and enough sleep. These aspects work together to improve an individual's general health, laying the groundwork for ulcer healing.

Essential Vitamins And Minerals For Ulcer Treatment

Nutrition is essential for ulcer management, and some vitamins and minerals are especially effective in promoting recovery. Vitamin A, which is renowned for its function in tissue healing, may help mend the damaged stomach or intestinal lining. Sweet potatoes and carrots are examples of vitamin A-rich foods that may be included in an ulcer rehabilitation diet.

Vitamin C is another crucial mineral with antioxidant capabilities that might help the immune system and heal ulcers. Citrus fruits, strawberries, and bell peppers are great sources of vitamin C.

Zinc, a mineral required for wound healing, is also useful in ulcer care. Foods that contain it include nuts, seeds, and legumes. These vitamins and minerals, when received via a well-balanced diet, help the body repair and rebuild damaged tissues, therefore promoting ulcer healing.

Detoxification For Ulcer Recovery: Cleaning The Body Naturally.

Detoxification, in the context of ulcer rehabilitation, is the act of removing toxins from the body to improve general health. While detox diets and cleanses are debatable, some lifestyle choices might naturally aid the body's detoxification functions.

Hydration is an essential part of detoxification. Drinking enough water helps to flush out pollutants and improves the general operation of biological systems. Herbal teas, especially those with anti-inflammatory characteristics, such as chamomile or ginger tea, may soothe the digestive system and assist in detoxification.

Including fiber-rich foods in your diet is another natural strategy to aid with detoxification. Fiber stimulates regular bowel movements, which helps to prevent toxins from building up in the digestive tract.

CHAPTER FOUR
Alternative Therapies: Acupuncture, Massage, And More

Alternative treatments provide additional options for those seeking holistic methods of ulcer repair. Acupuncture, an ancient Chinese therapy that involves inserting small needles into particular places on the body, has been studied for its potential to treat a variety of health issues, including ulcers. According to several research, acupuncture may help decrease ulcer-related discomfort and inflammation.

Massage therapy is another treatment option that may help people with ulcers. Gentle massages may assist to relax the muscles, decrease tension, and enhance blood circulation, all of which contribute to overall wellness. Individuals with ulcers should check with healthcare specialists before pursuing alternative remedies to verify compatibility with their treatment programs.

Navigating The Medication And Supplement Options

Medication and vitamins, when combined with holistic techniques, play an important role in ulcer management and treatment. Proton pump inhibitors (PPIs) and H2 blockers are often given to limit stomach acid production, hence alleviating ulcer symptoms and promoting healing.

Furthermore, certain supplements may be used in conjunction with conventional medical therapies. Probiotics, for example, promote the balance of healthy bacteria in the stomach, which may benefit the healing process. Individuals should speak with healthcare specialists before adding supplements to their routine to confirm their safety and efficacy.

Understanding the mind-body link and pursuing a holistic approach to ulcer treatment requires significant lifestyle changes. Individuals may improve their chances of recovering successfully from ulcers by addressing their physical, emotional, and psychological well-being. Balancing traditional medical treatments with alternative therapies, adequate diet, and mindfulness techniques results in a synergistic healing strategy that takes into account the complexities of the mind-body relationship in ulcer care.

Living with the constant fear of ulcers may be difficult, but taking a proactive approach via lifestyle changes can considerably help with long-term ulcer prevention. This includes not just individual efforts, but also developing a strong support structure, measuring progress, and celebrating milestones along the way to an ulcer-free life.

Lifestyle Changes For Long-Term Ulcer Prevention

Ulcers, whether gastric or peptic, are often caused by a mix of variables such as nutrition, stress, and lifestyle choices. Making conscious changes in these areas can help prevent and manage ulcers in the long run.

Dietary Adjustments

Diet is a key component in ulcer prevention. Avoiding hot and acidic meals might help soothe the stomach lining. Consuming more fiber-rich foods, such as fruits, vegetables, and whole grains, improves digestive health. Furthermore, eating a balanced diet ensures that the body gets the nutrients it needs to function properly.

Limiting caffeine, alcohol, and tobacco usage is critical since these chemicals may irritate the stomach lining and slow the healing process. Choosing smaller, more frequent meals over large, heavy ones can also reduce the digestive burden and help prevent ulcers.

CHAPTER FIVE

Stress Management

Chronic stress is a known cause of ulcer development. Meditation, yoga, and deep breathing exercises are all stress-reduction practices that may help you feel calmer. Creating a balance between work and personal life is critical, since overcommitment and an excessive workload may lead to increased stress.

Regular physical activity is another effective stress-management technique. Endorphins, the body's natural mood enhancers, are released during exercise and may help to counterbalance the negative effects of stress. Whether it's a brisk stroll, running, or participating in a favorite sport, including physical exercise in your routine benefits both your mental and physical health.

Building A Support System: Family, Friends, And Healthcare Professionals

The issues of ulcer prevention and treatment should not be taken on alone. Establishing a solid support system may give emotional, practical, and medical aid.

Family and friends.

Open communication with family and friends is crucial. Educating people about the disease, its causes, and the required lifestyle modifications helps build understanding and collaboration. Encourage loved ones to engage in dietary changes and stress-reduction exercises to create a supportive home atmosphere.

Social support is crucial for emotional well-being. Sharing ideas, worries, and accomplishments with family and friends may help to reduce the emotional toll of living with the continual fear of ulcers. Furthermore, their support might act as a motivator to stick to the recommended lifestyle adjustments.

Healthcare Professionals

Regular contact with healthcare specialists is crucial for ulcer prevention. Establishing a collaboration with an experienced healthcare team guarantees adequate monitoring, early intervention, and personalized instruction.

Routine check-ups, including endoscopies and imaging, enable healthcare specialists to analyze the stomach lining and spot any possible concerns early on. This proactive strategy is critical to good ulcer prevention. Furthermore, discussing symptoms, concerns, and progress with healthcare experts allows for any necessary revisions to the treatment plan.

In addition to medical specialists, consulting a registered dietitian or nutritionist may assist in building a personalized dietary plan that corresponds with individual health objectives and ulcer prevention requirements.

Tracking Progress: Monitoring and Adjusting Your Treatment Plan

Effective ulcer prevention requires consistent progress monitoring. This includes monitoring food patterns, stress levels, and general well-being. Keeping a diary of everyday activities, symptoms, and emotional states might give useful information.

Dietary Tracking

Keeping a food diary assists in identifying dietary triggers and trends that may lead to ulcer formation. Individuals who chronicle their meals, snacks, and drinks might identify particular items that cause symptom aggravation or alleviation. This information becomes a valuable tool for fine-tuning dietary decisions to improve ulcer prevention.

Stress And Emotional Wellbeing

Regularly monitoring stress levels and emotional well-being is also essential. A food diary may help you discover stresses, triggers, and coping strategies. Recognizing trends enables people to proactively address stresses and modify their stress management approaches.

Periodic self-assessments, such as anxiety and depression exams, give information on emotional health. When required, seeking the help of a mental health expert may be critical to general well-being and ulcer prevention.

CHAPTER SIX

Physical Activity And Lifestyle Habits

Tracking physical activity is essential for leading an active and healthy lifestyle. Setting realistic fitness goals and tracking progress helps people remain committed to regular exercise, which benefits both physical and emotional health.

Monitoring lifestyle factors, such as sleep patterns and hydration levels, rounds out the whole approach to progress monitoring. Quality sleep and sufficient hydration are critical components of ulcer prevention, and people may make changes depending on their monitoring results.

Celebrating Success: Obtaining And Maintaining Ulcer-Free Living

Acknowledging and applauding accomplishments on the path to ulcer prevention is critical for motivation and long-term commitment to a healthy lifestyle.

Small Victories.

Recognizing and applauding little accomplishments, such as adhering to a diet for a week or effectively managing stress at a difficult time, builds confidence and encourages beneficial habits. These tiny triumphs help to ensure the ultimate effectiveness of ulcer prevention.

Regular Check-Ins

Regularly reassessing objectives and changing the ulcer prevention strategy as required is an important part of long-term success. Celebrating success during these check-ins keeps people motivated and dedicated to their chosen path.

Conclusion: Adopting A Healthy, Ulcer-Free Lifestyle

To summarize, implementing lifestyle changes for long-term ulcer prevention is a multidimensional path that includes food changes, stress management, developing a strong support network, and constant self-monitoring. Engaging with healthcare experts, family, and friends builds a strong support network that improves the efficacy of ulcer prevention initiatives.

Individuals may avoid ulcers and live a better, more meaningful existence by measuring progress, appreciating victories, and having a proactive mentality. Finally, the path to an ulcer-free existence is an ongoing process of self-discovery, resilience, and dedication to well-being.